THE BETTER NECK BOOK

YOUR GUIDE TO NECK HEALTH

TANYA BELL-JENJE

BSC PHYSIO (UCT); MSC PHYSIO (WITS)

The Better Neck Book

Published by Groovi-Movements

Bryanston, South Africa

tanya@groovimovements.co.za

ISBN 978-0-7961-9409-1
eISBN 978-0-7961-9410-7

2 4 6 8 10 9 7 5 3 1

Layout by Boutique Books

Images courtesy Groovi Movements Exercise Software

Dedication

*For my husband Clem and children Paige
and Matt: Love you more than Salt*

Tanya Bell-Jenje is a South African physiotherapist with over 35 years of clinical experience. Tanya is actively practising as a healthcare practitioner in Johannesburg and is the director of both BRH Physiotherapists and Off Nicol Wellness Centre. She is recognised as one of the foremost experts in musculo-skeletal pain and has lectured at numerous conferences and workshops worldwide. Her interest in chronic pain and the use of patient empowerment through education, support, goal setting and functional exercise have made *The Better Back* and *The Better Neck* books a 'must read'.

CONTENTS

QUICK OVERVIEW AND TIPS

TIPS ON DEALING WITH NECK PAIN

- Serious injury is rare. Most people do recover within three months or less.

See more on
- Page 7: Dealing with neck pain

TIPS ON THE ANATOMY OF THE NECK

- The anatomy of your neck shows that your spine is flexible and strong.
- Our necks are designed for lots of movement, allowing us to turn and move our heads.

See more on
- Page 8 – 10: Understanding the anatomy

TIPS ON THE MECHANISMS OF PAIN

- A lot of chronic pain is mostly about brain sensitivity.
- Pain becomes less painful when we are confident that we are safe.
- Pain is influenced by our thoughts and emotions.

See more on
- Pages 11 – 13: The mechanisms of pain

TIPS ON X-RAYS, IMAGING AND MEDICATION

- Don't fixate on X-rays and scans that show changes in your spine. They usually have nothing to do with what you are feeling and are a normal part of ageing.
- Reduce your reliance on chronic medications.

See more on

- Page 14: How useful are X-rays, MRI scans, imaging and chronic medications?

TIPS FOR WHEN IN PAIN

- Bed rest can be more harmful than helpful, because it weakens the muscles that support the neck, back and body.
- Ideally, spend no more than a day or two in bed.
- Rest and get worse, or get active and recover.

See more on

- Page 15: When in pain, should I rest in bed?
- Page 17: When in pain, should I wear a neck collar?

TIPS ON WHEN TO SEE A DOCTOR

- When the neck pain is accompanied by another illness.
- When the pain is constant and does not seem to be related to or change with movement.
- When the pain follows a serious illness such as cancer.

See more on

- Page 18: When to see a doctor

TIPS ON MANAGING LESS SERIOUS SYMPTOMS

- Pain that is not there all the time is generally less serious.
- Sharp, catching pain that is always in one direction is too.

See more on
- Page 19: Less serious symptoms

TIPS ON FACTORS THAT MAKE NECK PAIN WORSE

- Manage and improve your general health where possible.
- Moving around reduces chronic neck pain.
- Improve your diet and nutrition and adopt a healthy lifestyle.
- Improve your sleep hygiene so that you average seven to eight hours of good sleep each night.
- Relaxation techniques help improve breathing, ease muscle tension and control feelings of stress and anxiety.
- Be conscious of your posture. Move every 20 minutes.

See more on
- Page 20 – 24: Associated factors

TIPS ON EXERCISE AND GOAL SETTING

- Motion is lotion. Lubricate and loosen those stiff joints and sore muscles.
- Develop exercise routines. Set realistic short- and long-term goals, and pace yourself to build up to a realistic exercise regimen.

- Follow the rehabilitation exercises prescribed by your physiotherapist.
- Discuss your fears and anxieties with your physiotherapist. Chatting to someone can help ease your worries. Stay motivated. A positive outlook is essential to speed up your recovery.

See more on

- Page 25 – 27: Exercise and goal setting

TIPS ON MANAGING DAILY LIFE

- Be conscious of how you position yourself at your desk, when driving and when sitting or standing.
- Make sure you sleep on a good quality mattress and comfortable pillow.
- Continue with the activities you enjoy, including sports.

See more on

- Pages 28 – 29: Managing daily life

TIPS ON MANAGING FLARE-UPS

- Flare-ups can happen. Be confident that the pain will settle down.
- Positive thoughts such as 'this will get better – it always does' will help
- Practise your relaxation techniques.

See more on

- Page 29 – 30: What to do about flare-ups

DEALING WITH NECK PAIN

Acute, recurrent and persistent neck pain is very common and is recognised as one of the leading causes of disability worldwide. Up to 70 percent of people will develop neck pain at least once during their lifetime[1]. In Southern Africa, seven percent of the population can experience neck pain at any given moment[2].

It can be very worrying when you develop neck pain, and at the outset the pain can be severe. Fortunately, serious injury or permanent damage is rare, and most people do get better. In fact, most neck injuries are not related to any specific abnormalities found in the structures of the spine[3]. Few people with neck pain have a disc problem or a trapped nerve.

Most people do recover from neck injury, with the help of their physiotherapist and other medical professionals. However, the most important person in this recovery process is you. The better you understand your condition and take an active role in managing it, the quicker and better you will recover. Current research supports a positive health approach to persistent pain. This encourages you to adapt and learn to self-manage your condition. It puts you in charge[4].

Positive health encourages high-quality, meaningful lives for people with chronic or persistent pain. Research shows that staying in bed, cancelling social activities or staying away from work are unhelpful and can, in fact, worsen your condition. There may be no cure for your condition, but with the right support you may find ways to manage pain so that life continues normally and successfully.

The Better Neck Book guides you on what to do and what not to do to help you adapt and get on the road to recovery. It educates you about neck pain while guiding you on ways to prevent further injury.

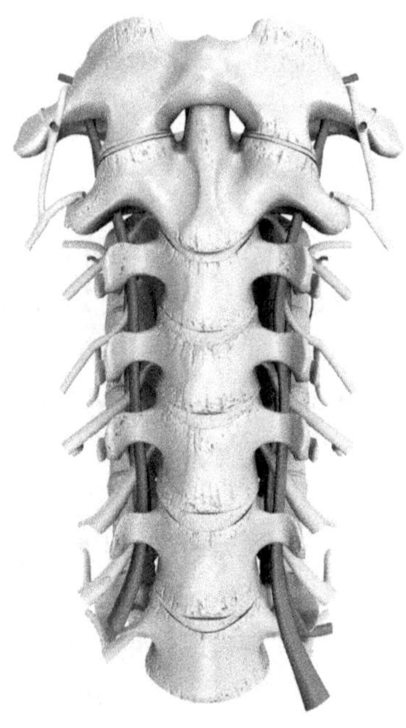

The neck or cervical spine is flexible and strong. It consists of seven cervical vertebrae and six intervertebral discs lodged between each vertebra, acting as shock absorbers. The cervical spine protects the spinal cord and has small holes in each vertebra through which the nerves to the shoulder, arms and hands run.

Our necks are designed for movement – lots of it – with most flexion, extension and rotation occurring at the top two vertebrae. This is to allow our heads to turn and move. The bones, ligaments, muscles and tendons support the weight of the head, which weighs between four and five kilograms.

The bones of the neck, or vertebrae, share the weight of the head between the discs at the front and the facet joints at the back of the vertebrae. This load-sharing is achieved thanks to the normal C curve shape of the neck, called a lordosis. We can lose this lordosis as a result of muscle spasm following an injury such as whiplash, or even from working in a sustained position, for example at our computer or on our smartphone. Losing the normal lordosis can overload some of the pain-sensitive structures, thereby causing neck pain. You may feel as if your head is too heavy and that the neck is unable to support its weight.

Twenty percent of the neck's stability can be ascribed to the bones and ligaments, and 80 percent to the neck muscles. This is an exciting fact, because it tells us that, if we strengthen the deep neck muscles, we can improve our neck control and reduce pain.

It is normal over time and as we age to see wear and tear, even bulging of some of the discs. This is simply a consequence of the neck doing its job. Often these discs bulge and cause no symptoms at all. But if the disc bulges and pushes onto a nerve, it can cause pain in the neck and even arm pain. What is interesting is that such pain is not usually permanent. As the bulging disc dehydrates and becomes smaller over time, it takes the pressure off the structures causing the pain[5].

The pain-generating joints at the back of the cervical vertebrae are called facet joints. A facet joint is similar to a knee or a hip joint. It has a capsule or sleeve surrounding it, with its own supporting ligaments and nerves. Just like a knee joint, these joints can become painful over time. Again, just like a knee or hip joint, we can learn to adapt and find positions and activities that do not aggravate the joint pain.

The deep stabiliser muscles of the neck are called the deep neck flexor and deep neck extensor muscles. They are also sometimes called the muscle sleeve of the neck.

These deep neck muscles work together to co-contract and provide joint control, optimising function during all the activities of daily living[6]. When you develop neck pain, the muscle sleeve switches off and doesn't function correctly. These muscles no longer provide control as they atrophy or waste away.

Often people describe that their head feels heavy and that they need to support it or hold it up. For this reason, we need to regain control of and strength in these muscles to improve your symptoms and get them back to the activities, sports and hobbies they enjoy.

Specific exercises of the neck, shoulder, upper back and scapula or shoulder blades will be of benefit to help you self-manage your chronic neck condition[7].

Different classifications or subgroups of neck pain exist. Some include neck pain with headache, neck pain because of whiplash injury, neck pain with mobility difficulties and neck pain with radiating pain[8,9]. Since there are different potential sources of neck pain, people present with a variety of symptoms. If you and your neighbour both have neck pain, the movements or positions that cause you pain may be helpful for them.

Also, the way you experience pain will be different to your neighbour's experience. You may describe your pain as a deep ache, whereas your neighbour may say it's like a sharp stab, or as if ants are running up and down their arm. Some people experience neck pain when reversing their car, while others may have pain when they extend their necks backwards, such as when looking up while working overhead.

Since no two people's symptoms are exactly the same, some of the treatment advice, management and rehabilitation need to be specifically prescribed for you. By understanding the anatomy and biomechanics of your cervical spine, we can guide you to avoid the aggravating positions and help you self-manage your chronic neck condition.

The natural history of neck pain is that only 20 percent of patients will recover within six weeks. Many patients go on to experience recurrent pain and disability within a year[10], and a number of factors have been identified as predictive reasons for why people develop chronic neck pain[11]. *The Better Neck Book* helps you to understand all the risk factors and guides you to better manage and improve your neck pain.

Chronic pain

Acute pain that lasts a few days or weeks is usually associated with tissue damage. Chronic or persistent pain is there for three months or longer, but tissue damage is not the main issue. After three to six months, most of the tissue healing that would have taken place already has. This means a lot of chronic pain is more about the sensitivity of the brain and the nervous system and less about tissue damage. Effectively, the brain produces an experience of pain that is out of proportion to the tissue damage that remains. Chronic pain can be weird and confusing. It is sometimes described as a complex witch's brew manufactured by the brain[12]. To better manage chronic pain, we need to retrain the brain and the sensitivity of the nervous system.

PAIN = ALARM but **PAIN ≠ HARM**

A common misconception is that if you feel pain, then harm or damage must be being done to your body's tissues. This is not the case. Pain is not a reliable sign of what is really going on. In fact, pain acts as an alarm. Sometimes, it's merely the brain being overprotective with nothing coming from the tissues at all. The good news is that we can retrain our overprotective pain system to be less protective. So, pain does not equal harm. Instead, it is a warning signal that tissue may be overstressed.

Sometimes, the pain system can malfunction, causing pain that is much more intense than it should be, or creating strange and unusual sensations. Awful pain does not mean you are in awful danger[13].

Pain is influenced by thought, emotion and movement

When you are fearful or anxious you can mistakenly believe that normal pulling or stretching sensations are pain. This means that you can become scared to move and your nervous system becomes so overactive that pain is produced too quickly and too severely. This hypersensitivity creates even more fear and then you become more and more afraid to move. This can turn into a vicious cycle until you avoid movement altogether and put yourself to bed for long periods. This is how pain interferes. It stops you from moving and doing things that are meaningful to you.

Your thoughts, fears and beliefs influence your pain experience. Feelings that cause you to be stressed or anxious increase your sensitivity to pain and make the pain last longer[14]. Uncertainty is another culprit that creates anxiety. This includes uncertainty about your diagnosis, your personal past experiences of pain, and concern about why the pain doesn't make any sense[15]. The good news is that educating yourself about your condition is the proven cure for uncertainty[16]. Sometimes, it helps to step back and review your life, asking yourself whether troubling events happened around the time your pain developed. For many, recognising the link between upsetting emotions and your chronic neck pain can be part of the healing process.

The brain can turn pain up and down

Pain is less painful when we are confident that we are safe. This was the conclusion of a famous study undertaken during World War II. It found that a wounded soldier's pain was reduced when he was removed from the frontline[17]. The brain can overfire signals, making pain more severe than it should be. On the other hand, it can also regulate pain downward. By identifying that your pain may be the result of your brain overfiring signals, you can switch your brain to regulate pain downward. Movement and exercise, along with learning about your pain, are two important ways to take control and manage it. Fear and anxiety have more power to aggravate pain than any other state of mind. A happy and confident brain intensifies danger signals less than an anxious, miserable brain[16].

Moving and exercising are healthy and help reduce hypersensitivity. The expression 'motion is lotion' describes how the muscles, nerves and joints love to move. Pain equals alarm and should be respected. But pain does not equal harm and should therefore not be feared. We need to use exercise and movement to help retrain the brain.

Understand and accept pain. Also accept that you can have flare-ups. Because your nervous system is hypersensitive, these will come along from time to time.

X-rays, MRI scans and other types of imaging?

Scans are helpful to diagnose certain spinal injuries, but only when combined with a detailed clinical assessment. Scans and other investigations often show false positives[3]. This means that someone who has changes on a scan may have no symptoms related to those changes at all. As we get older, it is appropriate for our bones and joints to show signs of aging. This is normal. Degenerative changes on X-rays do not mean you have damage or arthritis. For this reason, scans are no longer recommended unless one suspects it may change the management of your condition, for example if a fracture or infection is suspected[18].

An X-ray or scan may be called for to help your medical practitioner or physiotherapist prescribe the correct exercise and treatment management, but this should be done only when combined with a detailed clinical assessment.

Chronic medications?

Your general practitioner, neurosurgeon or orthopaedic surgeon may prescribe various medications to help manage your neck pain. Use the medication as prescribed – it may be necessary during the first few weeks after you develop neck pain. But, as your condition improves, you are likely to find yourself less reliant on medication. Discuss reducing your medication with the doctor who prescribed it. Prolonged use of medication, not to mention reliance on medication, is not recommended. Opioid medication is addictive and doesn't address the underlying causes of pain.

Some strong opioids commonly used in South Africa include morphine, fentanyl and oxycodone. Weaker opioids include codeine and tramadol. These so-called passive treatments have been linked to worsening disability, whereas active treatments such as exercising have been linked to decreased disability[19,20]. Many medications come with unwanted side effects and are not intended for prolonged use.

Should I rest in bed?

Years ago, people with neck or back pain were sent to bed for weeks or even months. This, we now know, is possibly the worst thing you can do[21]. Bed rest is more harmful than helpful, because it

- weakens the muscles that support the back, neck and body
- reduces bone density, which results in weaker bones (osteopaenia or osteoporosis)
- leads to depression and other emotional states of mind, such as feelings of hopelessness and despair that slow down the healing process and make you more sensitive to pain
- tends to progress conditions into a more permanent or chronic state
- is considered a passive treatment, which has been linked to increased disability[19]
- makes it difficult to get out of bed and get going again

It is recommended that you spend no more than a day or two in bed, at most. It is also important to be active as soon as possible after your acute injury, even if this means you manage only a short walk. Remember you have a choice: rest and get worse, or get active and recover. Stay physically active and continue with your normal everyday activities.

Should I stay away from work?

A positive health approach encourages you to maintain your normal social and work activities. Staying away from work promotes depression, reduced self-worth, financial strain and loneliness. You may need to miss a few days of work in the beginning, but the sooner you can return to your daily routine the better. Distractions are helpful and it is unlikely that your neck will be worse at work than at home.

Studies suggest that staying off work, generally not getting on with your life, and waiting for your next doctor's or physiotherapy appointment significantly delays your recovery. This could cost you your job and create stress and strain at home.

An imbalance between work and family time, high work stress or an unpleasant or hostile work environment have been linked to a high occurrence of neck pain[22]. It may be important for you to recognise associated stress and decide how you can manage or improve them.

If needed, a good option would be to ask your employer if you may perform lighter duties for a week or two, while you recover. Reduce the time your neck is in a sustained position or reduce the frequency that you move your neck into painful positions. Your physio- or occupational therapist will be able to advise and make recommendations to you and your employer.

Should I avoid family, friends and socialising?

This has been found to be one of the unhealthiest things you can do. Your family and friends may notice warning signs if you are not coping well. For example, you may be moody or tearful and display feelings of hopelessness. Identify these signs before it's too late. Try to approach your neck condition in a positive frame of mind. Discuss your fears with your family, friends or support group. Get out of bed and stay active. Read *The Better Neck Book* and stay in touch with family and friends.

Support from your family and friends as well as your community can be uplifting and positive. It will also take your mind off your condition and make you aware of the well- being of those around you.

Can I take medication?

Yes, by all means take medication for short-term pain relief to help with a flare-up of your neck condition or for headaches. Paracetamol and anti-inflammatories are helpful for these. Muscle relaxants may also help. But make sure it is safe for you to take anti-inflammatory medication. If you are asthmatic, pregnant or have a stomach ulcer, for example, their use is contraindicated. It is important to stay ahead of pain, instead of chasing it. For this reason, take the medication every four to six hours for the first three to seven days, as instructed. If needed, your doctor can prescribe something stronger, but this is usually not necessary.

Should I wear a neck collar?

It is not recommended that you wear a collar for an acute flare-up of neck pain, because this may slow down recovery. In fact, exercise programmes have proven to be more effective in reducing pain than immobilising your neck in a collar[7]. However, if you have nerve pain radiating down your arm, the short-term use of a collar, for no longer than a week, may help[9].

Some symptoms related to neck pain may need greater medical attention than self- management and exercise. See a doctor if:

- your neck pain gets worse, not better despite your following all the recommendations
- your neck pain is accompanied by illness
- your neck pain is accompanied by a persistent headache or one that gets worse
- you experience numbness, pins and needles or weakness in both arms and hands
- you are unsteady when walking or standing
- you experience dizziness that keeps getting worse or is accompanied by nausea or vomiting
- your pain is constant and does not seem to be related to or change with movement
- you are in pain following a serious illness like cancer

If you develop any of these symptoms, contact your doctor or physiotherapist immediately. But please, do not be overly concerned. Remember, neck pain is rarely the result of serious disease.

Do I need surgery to fix my neck?

Most neck pain improves without surgery. A few people may need surgery for intractable pain, nerve root pain, or muscle weakness in an arm[23]. A non-surgical approach is a better option because you take control and self-manage your condition. Surgery is not the treatment of choice for chronic pain. It is the last resort. And it is not a magic bullet: it does not address the complex nature of chronic pain. It comes with risks, enforces time off work, requires bed rest and is expensive[24]. Rehabilitation and exercise are prescribed after surgery, so the whole process may take even longer. Once operated on, you run a high risk of repeat surgery, especially if the principles contained in *The Better Neck Book* are not followed. Rather, follow these from the get-go and avoid surgery altogether.

Less serious, more common symptoms

- Neck pain after staying in one position for too long a time, for example when working at your computer, or when knitting or painting
- Sharp catching pain that is always in one direction or with the same movement
- Pain that is not there all the time or, if it constant, the intensity varies, depending on what activity you are doing
- Morning stiffness when you wake up but which tends to ease as the day wears on
- Headaches that seem to start in the neck and extend into the head, or even behind the eyes
- Neck pain and headaches that seem to be aggravated by stress
- Neck pain during a jarring activity such as jogging
- Neck pain and related pain after a whiplash injury

ASSOCIATED FACTORS

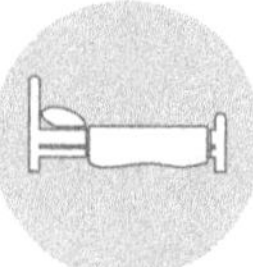 Develop good sleep habits/hygiene. Get a good mattress and pillow

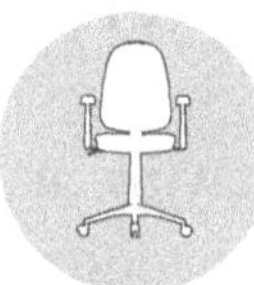 Correct ergonomics at desk

 Better management of co-morbidities (e.g. diabetes/hypertension)

 Stop smoking

 Relaxation/meditation to manage stress and anxieties. Fix the fixable

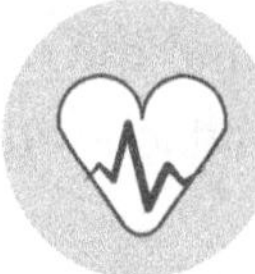 Regular prescriptive and cardiovascular exercise

 Weight loss/healthier eating habits. Reduce alcohol

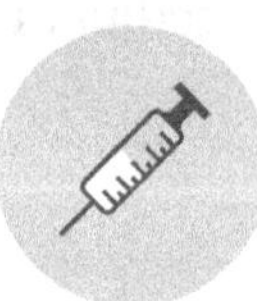 Avoid reliance on chronic pain medication but take when needed

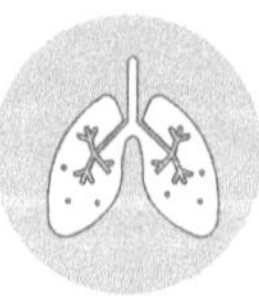 Diaphragmatic breathing is optimal

Factors that can aggravate neck pain

Factors associated with neck pain can either increase your risk of developing chronic neck pain or slow your recovery. These include:

- believing hurt means harm. Some people believe that they have a serious injury and will become disabled
- being trapped in a vicious cycle of fear of movement and avoiding it
- staying in bed for too long
- not taking responsibility for the condition; expecting others to sort it out
- withdrawing and becoming depressed, despondent and dejected[25]
- Believing you are unfairly treated at work, being stressed at work, or working in a hostile environment[22]

Fear of pain can be worse than the pain itself[26]. Being worried, anxious or afraid to move causes muscles to spasm or splint, and this often causes more pain than the actual neck pain itself[41].

People may tell you things that spark fear and anxiety, such as 'you can never exercise again', or 'you could be in a wheelchair soon'. Such damaging comments are almost always false. Ignore them and surround yourself with people who give you positive support. Trust the information in *The Better Neck Book* – it is based on the latest scientific research.

A positive, optimistic and motivated outlook has been shown to significantly improve outcomes in people with neck pain. Correct breathing and relaxation can help to reduce your stress and anxieties. Relaxation strategies will help to keep your mind from focusing on pain.

Underlying medical conditions

These can slow your healing time and increase your risk of developing neck pain. Underlying medical conditions include heart, lung and kidney disease, as well as diabetes, obesity, smoking and regular excessive alcohol intake. The best advice is to take an active role in managing these conditions.

Regular exercise that is planned and structured, along with a positive change to a healthier lifestyle, reduces the risk of death as a result of any of these diseases[27].

Obesity

Certain foods, such as those high in fat, or excessive eating and drinking of alcohol, not only create unhealthy excessive weight gains, but also increase the risk of many medical conditions such as hypertension (high blood pressure) and heart disease.

A large waist, or a high body mass index (BMI) is associated with diabetes, which also slows down healing. Being overweight increases the load on all your joints and is associated with more pain and poor functioning[20,28]. Excessive sugar intake is also associated with increased inflammation in the body, so keeping your intake of sugary drinks and snacks to a minimum will help reduce pain. A nutritious diet – both what you eat and drink – is essential to help reduce weight and improve your overall health.

Unhealthy sleeping habits

Experts recommend that you average seven to eight hours of good quality sleep a night. Poor, light or interrupted sleep is associated with an increase in the likelihood of developing chronic pain[29].

Prolonged or chronic use of sleeping tablets is not recommended as it is associated with other serious risk factors.

To improve your sleep hygiene, try to:

- get a good memory-foam pillow to reduce discomfort and to decrease snoring
- avoid using your cell phone or computer before going to bed, because the blue light emitted from the screen can cause insomnia
- use silicon earplugs to drown out external noises, such as your partner's snoring

Poor breathing

It is not healthy to breathe using your upper chest and not your diaphragm. This type of breathing is shallow and fast, and your neck muscles work hard to support it, resulting in persistent neck pain. This apical breathing pattern is common in people who are anxious or suffer from panic disorder[30], as well as in those with persistent neck or lower back pain[31]. Symptoms include shortness of breath, such as when climbing a flight of stairs, and rapid, irregular breathing. You may also experience muscle

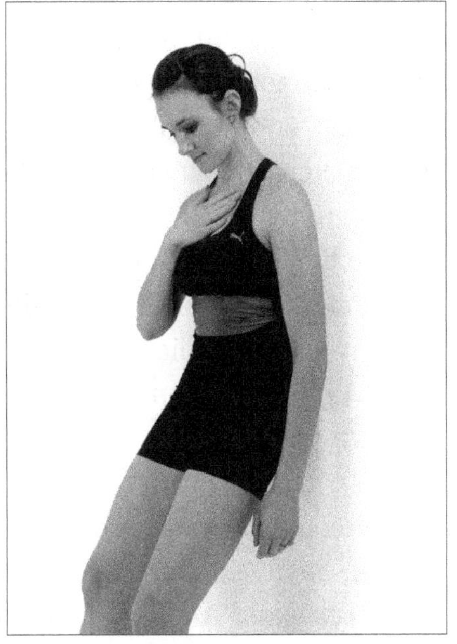

cramping, pins and needles in your hands and feet or problems with your circulation.

Correct breathing is called diaphragmatic breathing. As you breathe in, your lower ribcage expands and your tummy swells, so that you can inhale more air into your lungs[32,33]. With correct breathing, your upper chest remains relaxed, taking the strain off your neck muscles. Better oxygenation nourishes the brain and the muscles, while helping you to relax and sleep better.

Your physiotherapist will teach you to breathe correctly and give you exercises to strengthen your diaphragm. Relaxation techniques such as meditation, mindfulness and yoga, which use the correct breathing techniques, can help control feelings of anxiety, relieve muscle tension and help you manage your neck pain[6].

Hypermobility or joint laxity

People with genetically lax ligaments and other connective tissue tend to have more generalised joint and muscle pain than others. Joint hypermobility syndrome (JHS) runs in families and can present a complex and variable range of signs and symptoms. Between 19 and 30 percent of patients who attend physiotherapy or rheumatology clinics are hypermobile[34]. Your physiotherapist can assess whether you are hypermobile and prescribe exercises to help give you more joint control, if needed. If you do have JHS and it is an influencing factor in your chronic neck pain, try to wear Lycra gym pants that are too tight for you under your clothing[35]. This compression support can give you control around the trunk and pelvis, which can bring relief.

Better trunk control allows the neck muscles – which are trying to compensate by contracting or splinting – to relax, thereby relieving your neck pain. As with all the factors related to your persistent neck pain, your understanding of the condition, support from your physiotherapist and education on how to self-manage your condition will help you successfully manage your hypermobility and pain[36].

Poor posture

Standing or sitting in a slumped posture are examples of common abnormal sustained positions that can compress or overstretch parts of the spine and pelvis and cause pain. If you habitually adopt a pain-aggravating posture, your symptoms can be relieved just by changing to a pain-easing position[33]. Working in awkwardly sustained postures is an important risk factor to developing neck pain[25]. Your physiotherapist will teach you to correct or modify your posture in positions or places where you spend a lot of time. These may include sitting at your computer, standing and working overhead, or even working in your garden. Avoid staying in any single position for more than 20 minutes. Take frequent breaks when driving, get up from your desk and walk around, or do a few stretches. Specific exercises will help strengthen the core muscles of the neck and upper back to help you avoid sustained postures that provoke pain.

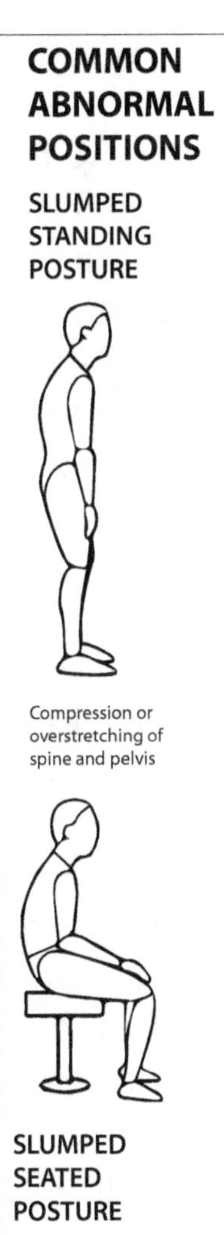

EXERCISE AND GOAL SETTING

How important is exercise?

Exercise is considered an active treatment. Being active reduces the risk of developing pain, while helping manage persistent neck pain[37,6]. Exercise also reduces chronic pain and fatigue, while decreasing depression and feelings of anxiety[38]. The concept of 'motion is lotion' reminds us how our bodies love to move for our health and well-being.

General exercises are essential for general health and fitness as well as for mental health. The World Health Organisation (WHO)[39] recommends at least 150 minutes of moderate exercise weekly. Regular physical exercise reduces the risk of stroke, heart disease, breast and colon cancer, diabetes and depression. It is essential for energy balance and weight control. It lubricates and loosens up stiff joints and muscles while releasing endorphins, our bodies' natural pain-relieving medication.

Light exercise includes activities such as walking the dog or walking to the shops. An example of moderate exercise would be mowing the lawn or attending a Pilates class. General exercise such as swimming or cycling places less load on the joints and muscles than others and may be more comfortable for you. While you recover, you may need to stay away from heavy-loading gym exercise such as weightlifting.

But, as you improve, heavy-loading exercises may be good for you, especially if this is something you either love or need to do to cope with lifting or other physical tasks.

Recommended exercises

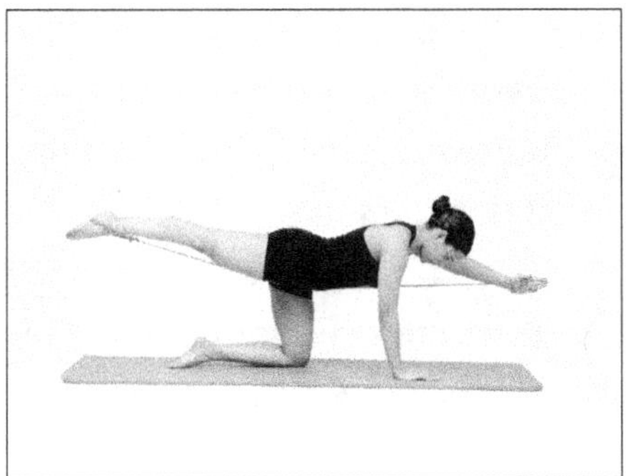

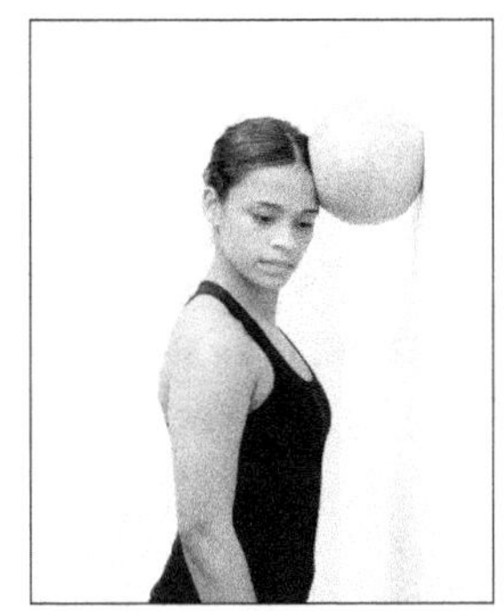

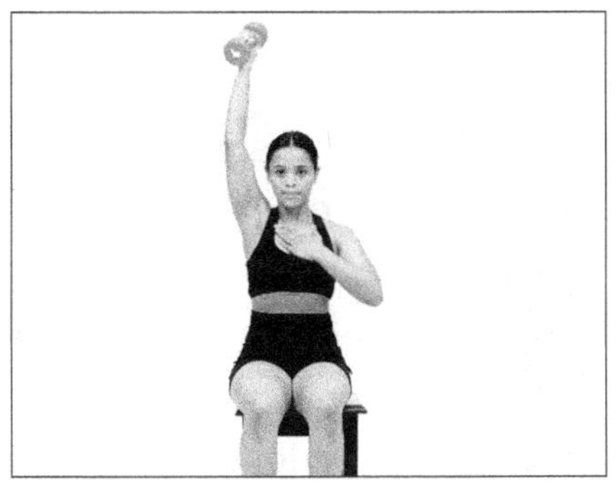

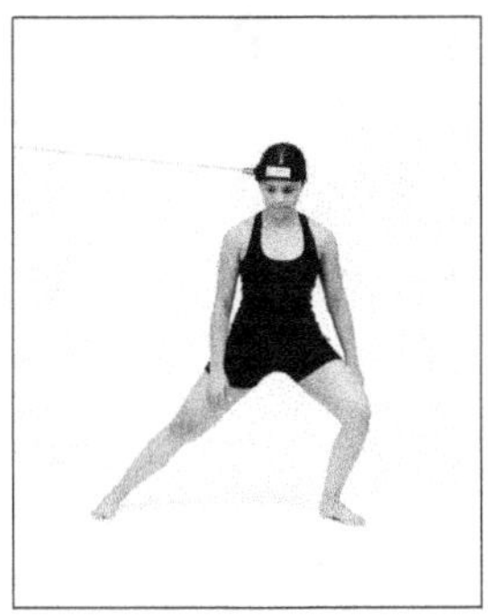

Positive movement means that you should move as if you are more comfortable than you really are[40]. Build up your confidence with whatever movement you can handle. Although this may seem like a lot of effort in the beginning, it is one of the best ways to self-manage your neck condition. Move and exercise in ways that are fun and pleasant. Recommended exercise options while the pain is still quite severe include swimming while breathing through a snorkel or attending an aqua-therapy or gentle yoga class. As you return to exercise, start slowly and do a little more each day so that you can see the progress you are making.

Specific exercises are needed to strengthen the deep neck muscles that surround the neck (core) to improve neck control and mobility and to reduce your neck pain[41]. Your physiotherapist will prescribe exercises to strengthen the muscles of your upper back, shoulders and scapula, among others. These will improve function by improving your strength, control, posture, flexibility and mobility[42,43,6].

Your physiotherapist will also teach you general exercises along with exercises specifically designed to strengthen your neck. This will improve your ability to go about your daily activities without serious pain.

Goal setting

It is important to perform your physical activities as well as your prescribed exercises consistently and regularly. Develop a routine and stick to it. If you have not been active until now, take the opportunity to improve your health and mobility with a new positive approach and a daily exercise regimen. Aim to do something active every day. Try to find an activity you enjoy. It is a lot easier to find motivation if you commit to a gym class or something like yoga. Join Park Runs or a walking club. Find an exercise buddy to do your exercise with at a set time or place. Set achievable goals such as joining a ten-kilometre community-organised event. Both short- and long-term goal setting can be very motivational. These options offer opportunities for positive social involvement that will help you feel optimistic and hopeful. Increase the challenge by modifying your goals to be more challenging as you get stronger. Ask your physiotherapist to help you set short- and long-term goals to reach your aims of being more active or of returning to activities you enjoy.

When should I start exercising?

The short answer is, as soon as you can. Exercise is essential to break the pain cycle. In fact, many people use exercise to successfully manage their pain[38,37]. Remember, if something hurts, it does not mean you are doing harm[44]. Pace yourself by developing a daily activity routine that is easily achievable. Sometimes, the toughest part is starting to exercise or move after a long break. But as soon as you see it is achievable in small progressive steps, you will be on your way. Depending on how your body responds, you can gradually increase or decrease the number of movements, distance or time.

You may experience some muscle aches as you start a new exercise. This is normal.

Understand and accept your pain and use exercise for effective pain relief. The sooner you start, the better.

The benefits of exercise and activity include:

- improved mental health and better coping skills to deal with pain
- feelings of optimism, hopefulness and enthusiasm
- less sensitivity to pain
- strengthening of specific muscles that support the whole of your spine
- better general fitness
- better general flexibility
- weight loss
- better sleeping patterns
- better overall health, as the heart and lungs get a good workout

HOW TO SET UP A HEALTHY WORKSPACE

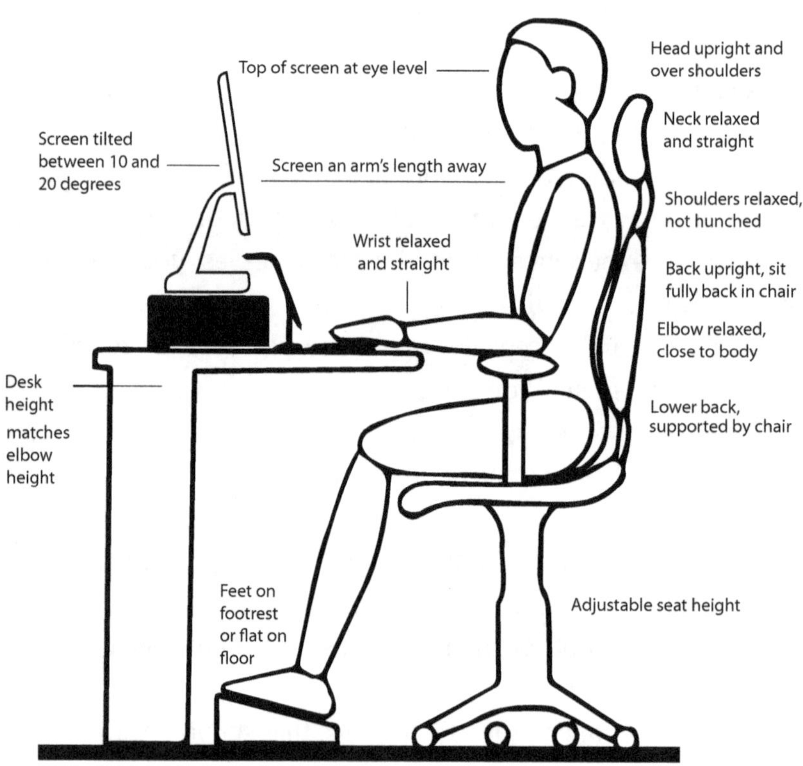

Working at my desk

If possible, use a good, adjustable ergonomic chair. Your head-on-neck position should form an ideal C curve to comfortably support the weight of the head. It is important that your upper back is not rounded or slumped, and that your chin does not poke forward, because this will overload the top of your neck. In this incorrect position your head may feel heavy and unsupported.

Your feet should rest on the floor with your knees slightly lower than your hips. The keyboard and monitor should be centred straight in front of you, so that your body does not rotate.

When sitting at your desk, your keyboard should be within easy range so that your forearms can rest on the desk when you type. The screen should be at eye height, at least an arm's length away from you.

Driving

Use a lumbar support cushion to ensure you are comfortable. Adjust the seat so that the headrest supports your neck. A useful pointer is that your hair should be in contact with the headrest.

Take frequent breaks – every hour or two – during long drives. Stop and get out of the car. Stretch and move around.

Sitting

Avoid staying in one position for too long. Prolonged sitting slows blood flow and restricts oxygen supply to your muscles.

If you are in a meeting, position yourself so that you are facing the speaker directly and so that your neck is not held in a sustained awkward or pain-provoking position.

We recommend two to three short breaks every hour. This will help your body recover from staying in one position for too long. Stretch and move around for a minute or two.

Sleeping

Wherever possible, make sure that you sleep on a good quality mattress with a firm base and comfortable pillow, ideally memory foam. When sleeping, your neck should be in a neutral position. The pillow should be as thick as the distance from the tip of your ear to the tip of your shoulder. If you sleep on your side, fold a small towel and place it under the pillow to achieve the correct height. We discourage sleeping on your stomach.

Sport

Continue to do the things that are fun and give you pleasure as much as you can. Depending on the sports activity, you may, in the short term, have to reduce either the frequency or intensity of the activity, or both. Ask your physiotherapist for guidance on goal setting for a realistic gradual return to the activities you enjoy.

KEEP THE JOURNEY POSITIVE

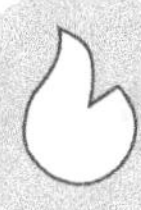 Don't panic. Flare-ups can happen from time to time

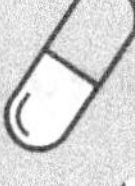 Use some meds in short term (Paracetamol, NSAIDs)

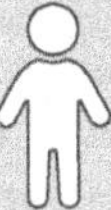 Physio to alleviate muscle spasms and guide you out of pain-provoking postures and positions

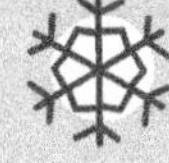 Ice first 72 hours

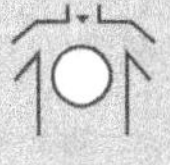 Correct your breathing

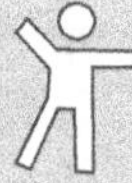 Specific stretches and core-strengthening exercises

 Assess ergonomics. Move every 20 minutes from desk or when driving

 Modify activities in the short term

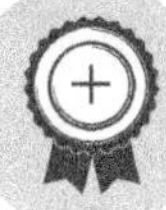 Remain positive. Stay as active as possible. Continue with life!

What do I do when my neck pain flares up?

As with many chronic medical conditions, neck pain may be with you on and off for life. The impact this has on your life depends on how you adapt and learn to self-manage your condition[4]. Part of self-management includes knowing what to do when you have a flare-up. The most important thing to do is not to panic. Understand that this can happen. Knowing this can greatly reduce the fear and anxiety associated with unexpected pain, which will help regulate the sensitised nervous system downwards[16].

A flare-up can happen unexpectedly for no known reason. It can be related to a sudden movement, illness, a change in the weather or a stressful event. Symptoms include muscle spasm, sharp pain, cramping or deep aches. Be confident that your pain will settle down. Positive thoughts such as 'this will get better, it always does' encourage a positive attitude that will help you cope with a flare-up much better[12].

Take control and manage the situation by:

- using medication for short-term pain relief. Paracetamol and anti-inflammatories may be helpful.
- applying an ice pack within the first 72 hours. We recommend that the ice is applied for 20 to 30 minutes, four or five times a day[45]. Thereafter, try to apply a form of heat such as a bean bag heated in the microwave oven or a hot water bottle.

- being kind to yourself. Create a safe, pleasant environment for yourself. Soak in a hot bath or go for a gentle massage. When your brain feels safe, the intensity of the pain goes down.
- gently performing stretches and the neck- or core-strengthening exercises your physiotherapist has taught you[6]. The motion-is-lotion principle reminds us that gentle exercise will lubricate the joints, ease muscle spasm and regulate the pain downwards[38,7].
- correcting your breathing to a deep, diaphragmatic pattern, and practising a relaxation technique.
- consulting with your physiotherapist if the pain is limiting your ability to self-manage your neck pain. It may be appropriate in an acute phase of pain for your physiotherapist to treat you with some hands-on treatment techniques to ease your muscle spasm and mobilise stiff joints[9].
- remaining positive and staying as active as possible as you continue with your life.

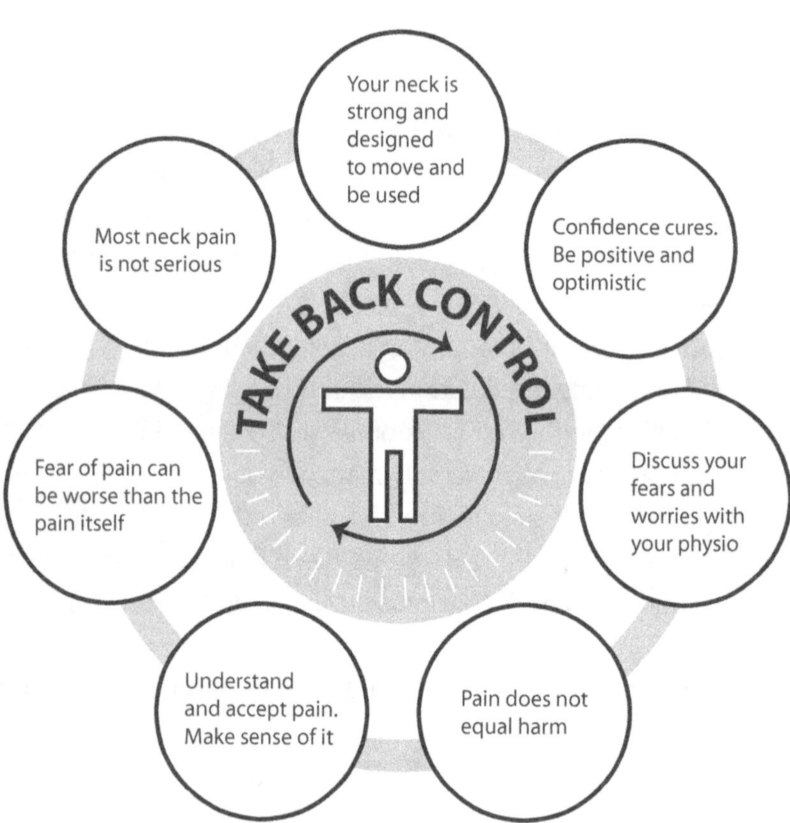

Your neck is strong and designed to move and be used
Most neck pain is not serious
Confidence cures. Be positive and optimistic
Fear of pain can be worse than the pain itself
TAKE BACK CONTROL
Discuss your fears and worries with your physio
Understand and accept pain. Make sense of it
Pain does not equal harm

- Most neck pain is not serious. Twenty percent of people with neck pain recover within six weeks.
- Pain does not equal harm. And awful pain does not mean you are in awful danger.
- A positive and optimistic outlook is essential to speed up your recovery.
- Don't fixate on X-rays and scans that show changes in your spine. They usually have nothing to do with how you feel and are a normal part of ageing.
- Education and confidence cures. Being informed builds confidence and this is one of the best ways to self-manage your condition.
- Pain is less intense when we know we are safe.
- Motion is lotion. Lubricate and loosen those stiff joints and aching muscles. Use exercise to regulate pain signals from the brain downwards.
- Develop exercise routines. Set realistic short- and long-term goals and pace yourself. Gradually build up how much you do and be realistic in your expectations.
- Follow the rehabilitation exercises your physiotherapist prescribes. Research shows they work.
- Improve your diet and nutrition, and adopt a healthy lifestyle. Go on a healthy or calorie-reduced eating plan if you need to lose weight.
- Practise relaxation techniques such as meditation, mindfulness or yoga to improve your breathing, and to bring feelings of fear and anxiety under control.

- Discuss your fears and anxieties with your physiotherapist. Chatting to someone will help you understand your condition and ease your worries. Stay motivated.
- Avoid bed rest that lasts more than a day or two. The sooner you get moving, the sooner you'll get better.
- Avoid staying in one position for too long. Take frequent breaks when driving or sitting.
- Stay in touch with your friends, family and community. Get back to work as soon as you can.
- Improve your sleep hygiene so that you get a good seven to eight hours' sleep a night.
- Manage and improve your general health wherever possible. A healthy, active lifestyle reduces chronic back and neck pain.
- Flare-ups do occur. But educating yourself about your condition by reading *The Better Neck Book*, adopting a healthier lifestyle and pacing yourself when doing regular exercise will reduce how often these come around, how intense they are and how long they last.
- Adopt a positive health approach. Take an active role in managing your condition. There may not be a cure, so learn to adapt and self-manage.
- Don't let your neck pain take over your life. Follow our guidelines so that life can continue normally and positively.

TAKE CONTROL.
YOU ARE IN CHARGE.
RETURN TO LIFE.

REFERENCES

1. Hoy, D., March, L., Woolf, A., Blyth, F., Brooks, P., Smith, E. et al., 2014, 'The global burden of neck pain: Estimates from the global burden of disease 2010 study', Annals of Rheumatic Diseases 73(7), 1309–1315. https://doi.org/10.1136/ annrheumdis-2013-204431

2. Basson, C. A., Olivier, B., & Rushton, A. (2019). Neck pain in South Africa: An overview of the prevalence, assessment and management for the contemporary clinician. *South African Journal of Physiotherapy*, *75*(1), 1–9. https://doi.org/10.4102/sajp.v75i1.1332

3. Huber M, van Vliet M, Giezenberg M, et al. Towards a 'patient-centred' operationalisation of the new dynamic concept of health: a mixed methods study. BMJ Open 2016; 5: e010091.

4. Nakashima, H., Yukawa, Y., Suda, K., Yamagata, M., Ueta, T., & Kato, F. (2015). Abnormal findings on magnetic resonance images of the cervical spines in 1211 asymptomatic subjects. *Spine*, *40*(6), 392–398. https://doi.org/10.1097/BRS.0000000000000775

5. Chiu CC, Chuang TY, Chang KH, Wu CH, Lin PW, Hsu WY. The probability of spontaneous regression of lumbar herniated disc: a systematic review. Clin Rehabil 2015; 29: 184–95.

6. Sterling M, de Zoete R, Coppieters I, Farrell S. Best evidence rehabilitation for chronic pain part 4: Neck Pain. *Journal Clinical Medicine. 2019;8(8):1219. doi:10.3390/jcm8081219*

7. Teasell RW, Mcclure J, Walton D, Pretty J, Salter, K, Meyer M. et al, 2010. A research synthesis of therapeutic interventions for whiplash-associated disorders (WAD): Part 2 interventions for acute WAD. Pain Research & Management: *The Journal of the Canadian Pain Society* 15(5), 295–304. https:// doi.org/10.1155/ 2010/106593

8. Haldeman, S., Johnson, C.D., Chou, R., Nordin, M., Côté, P., Hurwitz, E.L. et al., 2018, 'The global spine care initiative: Classification system for spine-related concerns', European Spine Journal 27(suppl 6), 889–900.

9. Blanpied, P.R., Gross, A.R., Elliott, J.M., Devaney, L.L., Clewley, D., Walton, D.M. et al., 2017, 'Neck pain guidelines: Revision 2017', Journal of Orthopaedic & Sports Physical Therapy 47(7), 511–512. https://doi.org/10.2519/jospt.2017.0507

10. Hush, J.M., Lin, C.C., Michaleff, Z.A., Verhagen, A. & Refshauge, K.M., 2011, 'Prognosis of acute idiopathic neck pain is poor: A systematic review and meta-analysis', Archives of Physical Medicine

and Rehabilitation 92(5), 824–829. https://doi.org/ 10.1016/j. apmr.2010.12.025

11. Walton, D.M., Carroll, L.J., Kasch, H., Sterling, M., Verhagen, A.P., Macdermid, J.C. et al., 2013, 'An overview of systematic reviews on prognostic factors in neck pain: Results from the international collaboration on neck pain (ICON) project', The Open Orthopaedics Journal 7(Suppl 4), 494–505. https://doi.org/10.2174/ 1874325001307010494

12. Ingraham P. Pain is weird https://www.painscience.com/articles/pain-is-weird.php

13. Moseley GL, Butler DS. Fifteen Years of Explaining Pain: The Past, Present, and Future. *J Pain*. 2015;16(9):807-813. doi:10.1016/j. jpain.2015.05.005

14. Karels CH, Bierma-Zeinstra SMA, Burdorf A, Verhagen AP, Nauta AP, Koes BW. Social and psychological factors influenced the course of arm, neck and shoulder complaints. *J Clin Epidemiol*. 2007;60(8):839-848. doi:10.1016/j.jclinepi.2006.11.012

15. Bunzli S, Smith A, Schütze R, Lin I, O'Sullivan P. Making sense of low back pain and pain-related fear. *J Orthop Sports Phys Ther*. 2017;47(9):628-636. doi:10.2519/jospt.2017.7434

16. Moseley GL. Whole of community pain education for back pain. Why does first-line care get almost no attention and what exactly are we waiting for? Br J Sports Med. 2018

17. Beecher HK. Relationship of significance of wound to pain experienced. JAMA. 1956 Aug;161(17):1609–1613. PubMed #13345630

18. Stochkendahl MJ, Kjaer P, Hartvigsen J et al (2017) National clinical guidelines for non-surgical treatment of patients with recent onset low back pain or lumbar radiculopathy. Eur Spine J 27(1):60–75.

19. Buchbinder R, van Tulder M, Öberg B, et al. Low back pain: a call for action. *Lancet*. 2018;391(10137):2384-2388. doi:10.1016/S0140-6736(18)30488-4.

20. Steffens D, Maher CG, Pereira LS, et al. Prevention of low back pain: a systematic review and meta-analysis. JAMA Intern Med 2016; 176: 199–208.

21. Almeida M, Saragiotto B, Richards B, Maher CG. Primary care management of non-specific low back pain: key messages from recent clinical guidelines. *Med J Aust*. 2018;208(6):272-275. doi:10.5694/ mja17.01152

22. Yang H, Hitchcock E, Haldeman S, et al. Workplace psychosocial and organizational factors for neck pain in workers in the United States. *Am J Ind Med*. 2016;59(7):549-560. doi:10.1002/ajim.22602

23. Eubanks J. Cervical Radiculopathy: Nonoperative Management of Neck Pain and Radicular Symptoms. *Am Fam Physician*. 2010;81(1):33-40. www.aafp.org/afp/2010/0101/p33.html.

24. Weinstein JN, Tosteson TD, Lurie JD, et al. Surgical versus nonoperative treatment for lumbar spinal stenosis four-year results of the Spine Patient Outcomes Research Trial. Spine 2010; 35: 1329−38.

25. Kim R, Wiest C, Clark K, Cook C, Horn M. Identifying risk factors for first-episode neck pain: A systematic review. *Musculoskelet Sci Pract*. 2018;33(November 2017):77-83. doi:10.1016/j.msksp.2017.11.007

26. Crombez G, Vlaeyen JWS, Heuts PHTG, Lysens R. Pain-related fear is more disabling than pain itself: Evidence on the role of pain-related fear in chronic back pain disability. *Pain*. 1999;80(1-2):329-339. doi:10.1016/S0304-3959(98)00229-2

27. Barry, V.W., Baruth, M., Beets, M.W., Durstine, J.L., Liu, J. and Blair, S.N. (2013), "Fitness vs. fatness on all-cause mortality: a meta-analysis", Progress in Cardiovascular Diseases, Vol. 56 No. 4, pp. 382-390.

28. Hartvigsen J, Hancock MJ, Kongsted A, et al. What low back pain is and why we need to pay attention. *Lancet*. 2018;391(10137):2356-2367. doi:10.1016/S0140-6736(18)30480-X.

29. Nijs J, Loggia ML, Polli A, et al. Sleep disturbances and severe stress as glial activators: key targets for treating central sensitization in chronic pain patients? *Expert Opin Ther Targets*. 2017;21(8):817-826. doi:10.10 80/14728222.2017.1353603

30. Yamada T, Inoue A, Mafune K, Hiro H, Nagata S. Recovery of Percent Vital Capacity by Breathing Training in Patients With Panic Disorder and Impaired Diaphragmatic Breathing. *Behav Modif*. 2017:014544551771143. doi:10.1177/0145445517711436.

31. Kolar P. Postural Function of the Diaphragm in Persons With and Without Chronic Low Back Pain. *J Orthop Sports Phys Ther*. 2012;42(4):352-362. doi:10.2519/jospt.2012.3830.

32. Mclaughlin L. Breathing evaluation and retraining in manual therapy. *J Bodyw Mov Ther*. 2009;13:276-282. doi:10.1016/j.jbmt.2009.01.005.

33. O'Sullivan PB, Beales DJ. Diagnosis & classification of pelvic girdle disorders – Part 1: A mechanism based approach within a biopsychosocial framework. Manual Therapy 2007; 12: 86-97.

34. Connelly, Emma et al. 'A Study Exploring the Prevalence of Joint Hypermobility Syndrome in Patients Attending a Musculoskeletal Triage Clinic'. 1 Jan. 2015 : 43 – 53.

35. Bluestein LS. Pain Management in Patients With Hypermobility Disorders. *Top Pain Manag*. 2017;32(12):1-10. doi:10.1097/01. tpm.0000521090.64732.c6

36. Terry RH, Palmer ST, Rimes KA, Clark CJ, Simmonds J V., Horwood JP. Living with joint hypermobility syndrome: Patient experiences of diagnosis, referral and self-care. *Fam Pract*. 2015;32(3):354-358. doi:10.1093/fampra/cmv026.

37. Palmlöf L, Holm LW, Alfredsson L, Magnusson C, Vingård E, Skillgate E. The impact of work related physical activity and leisure physical activity on the risk and prognosis of neck pain - A population based cohort study on workers. *BMC Musculoskelet Disord*. 2016;17(1):1-11. doi:10.1186/s12891-016-1080-1

38. Polaski AM, Phelps AL, Kostek MC, Szucs KA, Kolber BJ. Exercise-induced hypoalgesia: A meta-analysis of exercise dosing for the treatment of chronic pain. *PLoS One*. 2019;14(1):e0210418. doi:10.1371/journal.pone.0210418

39. World Health Organisation (2010), Prevalence of Insufficient Physical Activity, WHO Press, Geneva, available at: www.who.int/gho/ncd/risk_factors/physical_activity_text/en/

40. Hargrove T. www.bettermovement.org [Internet]. Why Your Body is a Hypocrite; 2017

41. Shahidi B, Curran-Everett D, Maluf KS. Psychosocial, Physical, and Neurophysiological Risk Factors for Chronic Neck Pain: A Prospective Inception Cohort Study. *J Pain*. 2015;16(12):1288-1299. doi:10.1016/j.jpain.2015.09.002

42. Cools AMJ, Struyf F, De Mey K, Maenhout A, Castelein B, Cagnie B. Rehabilitation of scapular dyskinesis: from the office worker to the elite overhead athlete. *Br J Sports Med*. 2014;48(8):692-697. doi:10.1136/bjsports-2013-092148

43. Gross AR, Paquin JP, Dupont G, Blanchette S, Lalonde P, Cristie T. et al, 2016. Exercises for mechanical neck disorders: A Cochrane review update, *Manual Therapy* 24, 25–45.

44. Geneen LJ, More RA, Clarke C, Martin D, Colvin LA, Smith BH. Physical activity and exercise for chronic pain in adults. J Sociol. 2017;(1):135-139.

45. Geneen LJ, More RA, Clarke C, Martin D, Colvin LA, Smith BH. Physical activity and exercise for chronic pain in adults. *J Sociol*. 2017;(1):135-139.

46. Guillot, X., Tordi, N., Mourot, L., Demougeot, C., Dugué, B., Prati, C., & Wendling, D. (2014). Cryotherapy in inflammatory rheumatic diseases: A systematic review. In *Expert Review of Clinical Immunology* (Vol. 10, Issue 2, pp. 281–294). Taylor & Francis. https://doi.org/10.158 6/1744666X.2014.870036